*To come to be
you must have a vision of being,
a dream, a purpose, a principle.
You will become what your vision is.*

Peter Nivio Zarlenga

Copyright Page:

So, I said to myself © Copyright 2020
Leslie Lindsey Davis

All rights reserved. No part of this publication may be reproduced, distributed or transmitted in any form or by any means, including photocopying, recording, or other electronic or mechanical methods, without the prior written permission of the publisher, except in the case of brief quotations embodied in critical reviews and certain other noncommercial uses permitted by copyright law. Although the author and publisher have made every effort to ensure that the information in this book was correct at press time, the author and publisher do not assume and hereby disclaim any liability to any party for any loss, damage, or disruption caused by errors or omissions, whether such errors or omissions result from negligence, accident, or any other cause. Adherence to all applicable laws and regulations, including international, federal, state and local governing professional licensing, business practices, advertising, and all other aspects of doing business in the US, Canada or any other jurisdiction is the sole responsibility of the reader and consumer. Neither the author nor the publisher assumes any responsibility or liability whatsoever on behalf of the consumer or reader of this material. Any perceived slight of any individual or organization is purely unintentional. The resources in this book are provided for informational purposes only and should not be used to replace the specialized training and professional judgment of a health care or mental health care professional. Neither the author nor the publisher can be held responsible for the use of the information provided within this book. Please always consult a trained professional before making any decision regarding treatment of yourself or others.

For
more information, email leslie@youcanteatlove.com
ASBN: 9798563952225
ISBN: 9781736232217

So, I said to myself...

A place to have a conversation with the most important person in your world...YOU

Have you ever wished you had someone you could talk to who would never get tired of listening? I've discovered some of the deepest and most meaningful conversations I can have are those I have with myself. I can tell myself anything and not be afraid of judgment.

This is your chance to have a conversation with yourself and discover who you really are. Be brave, be honest, be kind. On these pages talk to yourself just as you would talk to your very best friend in the whole wide world and listen as your bff talks to you.

At the beginning of the week, you'll have a chance to write down what you are going to focus on.
At the end of the week, you can tell your bff how it went.

Each day, share your celebrations (big and small), the great choices you made, and how you were kind to yourself. Your bff is just curious about what might be on your mind or why you made some of the choices you made. You even have several pages to just talk to your bff and reflect on what is going on in your world.

Date

• •

"To begin, begin."
— William Wordsworth

*"Not every week starts on a Sunday.
You do you and begin where you begin."*
— Leslie Lindsey Davis

"You've got to know yourself so you can at last be yourself."

D.H. Lawrence

Week 1

So, I said to myself...

...these are the three things I want to focus on this week and why.

Jan Feb Mar Apr May June July Aug Sept Oct Nov Dec
1 2 3 4 5 6 7 8 9 10 11 12 13 14 15 16 17 18 19 20 21 22 23 24 25 26 27 28 29 30 31

So, I said to myself, "guess what I celebrated!"

Great choices I made:

How I was kind to myself:

I'm just curious, if you could do one thing differently, what would you do?

Go on, I'm listening...

"Your time is limited, so don't waste it living someone else's life."
Steve Jobs

Jan Feb Mar Apr May June July Aug Sept Oct Nov Dec
1 2 3 4 5 6 7 8 9 10 11 12 13 14 15 16 17 18 19 20 21 22 23 24 25 26 27 28 29 30 31

So, I said to myself, "guess what I celebrated!"

Great choices I made:

How I was kind to myself:

I'm just curious, what makes you smile?

Go on, I'm listening...

"On a calm sea every man is a pilot."

English Proverb

Jan Feb Mar Apr May June July Aug Sept Oct Nov Dec
1 2 3 4 5 6 7 8 9 10 11 12 13 14 15 16 17 18 19 20 21 22 23 24 25 26 27 28 29 30 31

So, I said to myself, "guess what I celebrated!"

Great choices I made:

How I was kind to myself:

I'm just curious, you doing ok?

Go on, I'm listening...

"Make the most of yourself, for that is all there is of you."
Ralph Waldo Emerson

Jan Feb Mar Apr May June July Aug Sept Oct Nov Dec
1 2 3 4 5 6 7 8 9 10 11 12 13 14 15 16 17 18 19 20 21 22 23 24 25 26 27 28 29 30 31

So, I said to myself, "guess what I celebrated!"

Great choices I made:

How I was kind to myself:

I'm just curious, what are you grateful for?

Go on, I'm listening...

Jan Feb Mar Apr May June July Aug Sept Oct Nov Dec
1 2 3 4 5 6 7 8 9 10 11 12 13 14 15 16 17 18 19 20 21 22 23 24 25 26 27 28 29 30 31

So, I said to myself, "guess what I celebrated!"

Great choices I made:

How I was kind to myself:

I'm just curious, what do you love the most about yourself?

Go on, I'm listening...

"To enjoy life we must touch much of it lightly."

Voltaire (Francois-Marie Arounet)

Jan Feb Mar Apr May June July Aug Sept Oct Nov Dec
1 2 3 4 5 6 7 8 9 10 11 12 13 14 15 16 17 18 19 20 21 22 23 24 25 26 27 28 29 30 31

So, I said to myself, "guess what I celebrated!"

Great choices I made:

How I was kind to myself:

I'm just curious, what is your favorite part of your day?

Go on, I'm listening...

"Go out as far as you can and start from there."
Albert Enstein

Jan Feb Mar Apr May June July Aug Sept Oct Nov Dec

1 2 3 4 5 6 7 8 9 10 11 12 13 14 15 16 17 18 19 20 21 22 23 24 25 26 27 28 29 30 31

So, I said to myself, "guess what I celebrated!"

Great choices I made:

How I was kind to myself:

I'm just curious, what is your super power and how do you use it?

Go on, I'm listening...

"Courage is the master of fear, not the absence of fear."
Mark Twain

*"So", I asked myself,
"How was your week?"*

My quote for next week:

Week 2

So, I said to myself...

...these are the three things I want to focus on this week and why.

Jan Feb Mar Apr May June July Aug Sept Oct Nov Dec

1 2 3 4 5 6 7 8 9 10 11 12 13 14 15 16 17 18 19 20 21 22 23 24 25 26 27 28 29 30 31

So, I said to myself, "guess what I celebrated!"

Great choices I made:

How I was kind to myself:

I'm just curious, what is your super power and how do you use it?

Go on, I'm listening...

"The most wasted day of all is that on which we have not laughed."
Sebastien de Chamfort

Jan Feb Mar Apr May June July Aug Sept Oct Nov Dec
1 2 3 4 5 6 7 8 9 10 11 12 13 14 15 16 17 18 19 20 21 22 23 24 25 26 27 28 29 30 31

So, I said to myself, "guess what I celebrated!"

Great choices I made:

How I was kind to myself:

I'm just curious, what is your super power and how do you use it?

Go on, I'm listening...

"To conquer oneself is a greater task than conquering others."
Buddha

Jan Feb Mar Apr May June July Aug Sept Oct Nov Dec
1 2 3 4 5 6 7 8 9 10 11 12 13 14 15 16 17 18 19 20 21 22 23 24 25 26 27 28 29 30 31

So, I said to myself, "guess what I celebrated!"

Great choices I made:

How I was kind to myself:

I'm just curious, what is your super power and how do you use it?

Go on, I'm listening...

"The truth lies in a man's dreams."

Miguel de Cervantes

Jan Feb Mar Apr May June July Aug Sept Oct Nov Dec
1 2 3 4 5 6 7 8 9 10 11 12 13 14 15 16 17 18 19 20 21 22 23 24 25 26 27 28 29 30 31

So, I said to myself, "guess what I celebrated!"

Great choices I made:

How I was kind to myself:

I'm just curious, what is your super power and how do you use it?

Go on, I'm listening...

"Don't threaten me with love, baby. Let's just go walking in the rain."
Billie Holliday

Jan Feb Mar Apr May June July Aug Sept Oct Nov Dec
1 2 3 4 5 6 7 8 9 10 11 12 13 14 15 16 17 18 19 20 21 22 23 24 25 26 27 28 29 30 31

So, I said to myself, "guess what I celebrated!"

Great choices I made:

How I was kind to myself:

I'm just curious, what is your super power and how do you use it?

Go on, I'm listening...

"Fill your paper with the breathings of your heart."

William Wordsworth

Jan Feb Mar Apr May June July Aug Sept Oct Nov Dec
1 2 3 4 5 6 7 8 9 10 11 12 13 14 15 16 17 18 19 20 21 22 23 24 25 26 27 28 29 30 31

So, I said to myself, "guess what I celebrated!"

Great choices I made:

How I was kind to myself:

I'm just curious, what is your super power and how do you use it?

Go on, I'm listening...

"Be kind, for everyone you meet is fighting a hard battle."

Philo of Alexandria

Jan Feb Mar Apr May June July Aug Sept Oct Nov Dec
1 2 3 4 5 6 7 8 9 10 11 12 13 14 15 16 17 18 19 20 21 22 23 24 25 26 27 28 29 30 31

So, I said to myself, "guess what I celebrated!"

Great choices I made:

How I was kind to myself:

I'm just curious, what is your super power and how do you use it?

Go on, I'm listening...

"There is more to life than increasing its speed."

Mohandas K. (Mahatma) Gandhi

"So", I asked myself, "How was your week?"

My quote for next week:

Week 3

So, I said to myself...

...these are the three things I want to focus on this week and why.

Time to reorder *So, I said to myself...*

Jan Feb Mar Apr May June July Aug Sept Oct Nov Dec

1 2 3 4 5 6 7 8 9 10 11 12 13 14 15 16 17 18 19 20 21 22 23 24 25 26 27 28 29 30 31

So, I said to myself, "guess what I celebrated!"

Great choices I made:

How I was kind to myself:

I'm just curious, what is your super power and how do you use it?

Go on, I'm listening...

"I have measured out my life with coffee spoons."
T.S. Eliot

Jan Feb Mar Apr May June July Aug Sept Oct Nov Dec
1 2 3 4 5 6 7 8 9 10 11 12 13 14 15 16 17 18 19 20 21 22 23 24 25 26 27 28 29 30 31

So, I said to myself, "guess what I celebrated!"

Great choices I made:

How I was kind to myself:

I'm just curious, what is your super power and how do you use it?

Go on, I'm listening...

"Find out who you are and do it on purpose."

Dolly Parton

Jan Feb Mar Apr May June July Aug Sept Oct Nov Dec
1 2 3 4 5 6 7 8 9 10 11 12 13 14 15 16 17 18 19 20 21 22 23 24 25 26 27 28 29 30 31

So, I said to myself, "guess what I celebrated!"

Great choices I made:

How I was kind to myself:

I'm just curious, what is your super power and how do you use it?

Go on, I'm listening...

"Each man's life represents a road toward himself."

Hermann Hesse

Jan Feb Mar Apr May June July Aug Sept Oct Nov Dec
1 2 3 4 5 6 7 8 9 10 11 12 13 14 15 16 17 18 19 20 21 22 23 24 25 26 27 28 29 30 31

So, I said to myself, "guess what I celebrated!"

Great choices I made:

How I was kind to myself:

I'm just curious, what is your super power and how do you use it?

Go on, I'm listening...

"I wasn't searching for something or someone...
I was searching for me."

Carrie Bradshaw, *Sex and the City*

Jan Feb Mar Apr May June July Aug Sept Oct Nov Dec
1 2 3 4 5 6 7 8 9 10 11 12 13 14 15 16 17 18 19 20 21 22 23 24 25 26 27 28 29 30 31

So, I said to myself, "guess what I celebrated!"

Great choices I made:

How I was kind to myself:

I'm just curious, what is your super power and how do you use it?

Go on, I'm listening...

"A person often meets his destiny on a road he took to avoid it."

Jean de la Fontaine

Jan Feb Mar Apr May June July Aug Sept Oct Nov Dec
1 2 3 4 5 6 7 8 9 10 11 12 13 14 15 16 17 18 19 20 21 22 23 24 25 26 27 28 29 30 31

So, I said to myself, "guess what I celebrated!"

Great choices I made:

How I was kind to myself:

I'm just curious, what is your super power and how do you use it?

Go on, I'm listening...

"There is only one corner of the universe you can be certain of improving, and that's your own self."

Aldous Huxley

"So", I asked myself,
"How was your week?"

My quote for next week:

Week 4

So, I said to myself...

...these are the three things I want to focus on this week and why.

Time to reorder *So, I said to myself...*

Jan Feb Mar Apr May June July Aug Sept Oct Nov Dec
1 2 3 4 5 6 7 8 9 10 11 12 13 14 15 16 17 18 19 20 21 22 23 24 25 26 27 28 29 30 31

So, I said to myself, "guess what I celebrated!"

Great choices I made:

How I was kind to myself:

I'm just curious, if you could do one thing differently, what would you do?

Go on, I'm listening...

"All the wonders you seek are within yourself."

Thomas Browne

Jan Feb Mar Apr May June July Aug Sept Oct Nov Dec
1 2 3 4 5 6 7 8 9 10 11 12 13 14 15 16 17 18 19 20 21 22 23 24 25 26 27 28 29 30 31

So, I said to myself, "guess what I celebrated!"

Great choices I made:

How I was kind to myself:

I'm just curious, if you could do one thing differently, what would you do?

Go on, I'm listening...

"I long, as does every human being,
to be at home where ever I find myself."

Maya Angelou

Jan Feb Mar Apr May June July Aug Sept Oct Nov Dec
1 2 3 4 5 6 7 8 9 10 11 12 13 14 15 16 17 18 19 20 21 22 23 24 25 26 27 28 29 30 31

So, I said to myself, "guess what I celebrated!"

Great choices I made:

How I was kind to myself:

I'm just curious, if you could do one thing differently, what would you do?

Go on, I'm listening...

"You're never to old to set a new goal or to dream a new dream."
C.S. Lewis

Jan Feb Mar Apr May June July Aug Sept Oct Nov Dec
1 2 3 4 5 6 7 8 9 10 11 12 13 14 15 16 17 18 19 20 21 22 23 24 25 26 27 28 29 30 31

So, I said to myself, "guess what I celebrated!"

Great choices I made:

How I was kind to myself:

I'm just curious, if you could do one thing differently, what would you do?

Go on, I'm listening...

"Act as if what you do makes a difference. It does."

William James

Jan Feb Mar Apr May June July Aug Sept Oct Nov Dec
1 2 3 4 5 6 7 8 9 10 11 12 13 14 15 16 17 18 19 20 21 22 23 24 25 26 27 28 29 30 31

So, I said to myself, "guess what I celebrated!"

Great choices I made:

How I was kind to myself:

I'm just curious, if you could do one thing differently, what would you do?

Go on, I'm listening...

"Just don't give up trying to do what you really want to do.
Where there is love and inspiration, I don't think you can go wrong."

Ella Fitzgerald

Jan Feb Mar Apr May June July Aug Sept Oct Nov Dec
1 2 3 4 5 6 7 8 9 10 11 12 13 14 15 16 17 18 19 20 21 22 23 24 25 26 27 28 29 30 31

So, I said to myself, "guess what I celebrated!"

Great choices I made:

How I was kind to myself:

I'm just curious, if you could do one thing differently, what would you do?

Go on, I'm listening...

"Believe you can and you're halfway there."
Theodore Roosevelt

Jan Feb Mar Apr May June July Aug Sept Oct Nov Dec
1 2 3 4 5 6 7 8 9 10 11 12 13 14 15 16 17 18 19 20 21 22 23 24 25 26 27 28 29 30 31

So, I said to myself, "guess what I celebrated!"

Great choices I made:

How I was kind to myself:

I'm just curious, if you could do one thing differently, what would you do?

Go on, I'm listening...

"If people are doubting how far you can go,
go so far that you can't hear them anymore."

Michele Ruiz

So, I asked myself, "How was your week?"

My quote for next week:

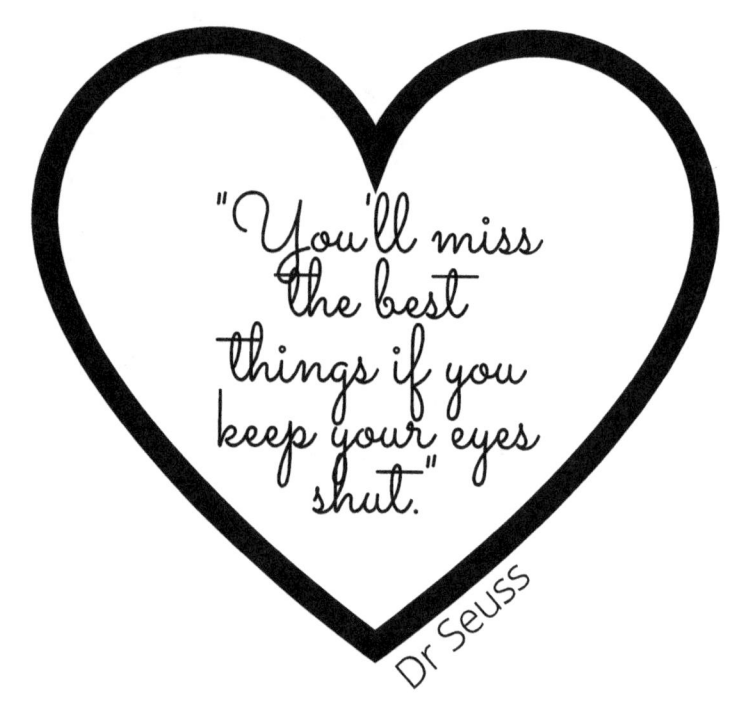

"You'll miss the best things if you keep your eyes shut."
Dr Seuss

I hope you've enjoyed your conversations with the most interesting human in the world, yourself. You can find this journal and more information at
www.joyandelephants.com
or hop over to the Facebook page
Joy and Elephants and chat.
I would love to hear from you.
Leslie Lindsey Davis

www.ingramcontent.com/pod-product-compliance
Lightning Source LLC
Chambersburg PA
CBHW070917080526
44589CB00013B/1336